E.COLI

THE KNOWN REMEDY FOR E.COLI INFECTION

DR.SCARLETT INGRAM

Contents

CHAPTER ONE 3

INTODUCTION 3

Symptoms and signs...7

What does E. Coli appear like?...7

How many lines of E. Coli motive diarrhea? 8

How does E. Coli make you ill?...9

Who can get inflamed with E. Coli? 10

Reasons 11

CHAPTER TWO 13

How is an E. Coli infection diagnosed?.......................15

What steps are worried in getting a stool pattern to my healthcare provider?..15

Some desired commands for gathering a stool sample at domestic consist of: 16

Whilst will i get the results once more from my stool pattern? 17

Treatments...18

Chance factors 20

Complications...22

CHAPTER THREE 23

Prevention..23

Volatile meals...23

Keep away from pass-infection.............................25

CONCLUSION..26

THE END...29

CHAPTER ONE

INTODUCTION

Escherichia coli (E. Coli) bacteria normally live within the intestines of healthy human beings and animals. Maximum types of E. Coli are harmless or purpose in particular brief diarrhea. However some strains, collectively with E. Coli O157:H7, can purpose excessive stomach cramps, bloody diarrhea and vomiting.

You may be uncovered to E. Coli from inflamed water or food — specifically uncooked veggies and undercooked floor beef. Healthful adults typically get over infection with E. Coli O157:H7 inside every week. More youthful kids and older adults have a extra threat of developing a lifestyles-threatening shape of kidney failure.

E. Coli normally lives for your intestines. Maximum lines are usually innocent. A few lines motive diarrhea/bloody diarrhea, vomiting and stomach pains and cramps. One strain can lead to kidney failure if now not well controlled. Ingesting infected meals is the maximum common way to get an E. Coli infection. The majority get better within in step with week with out medicines.

Escherichia coli (E. Coli) is a bacteria that normally lives in the intestines of every healthy human beings and animals. In maximum instances, this micro organism is harmless. It helps digest the meals you devour. But, high quality lines of E. Coli can cause signs and symptoms which include diarrhea, belly pain and cramps and coffee-grade fever. A few E. Coli infections may be dangerous.

E. Coli (Escherichia coli), is a type of bacteria that generally lives to your intestines. It's moreover determined inside the intestine of some animals.

Most forms of E. Coli are harmless and even assist preserve your digestive tract healthy. However a few lines can reason diarrhea in case you consume infected meals or drink fouled water.

Whilst plenty of us companion E. Coli with food poisoning, you can moreover get pneumonia and urinary tract infections from brilliant types of the micro organism. In truth, 75% to 95% of urinary tract infections are due to E. Coli. E.Coli is a everyday resident of the bowel, it really is the way it makes it manner to the urinary tract.

A few versions of E. Coli make you unwell via making a toxin referred to as Shiga. This toxin damages the liner of your gut. The lines of E. Coli that make the toxin are now and again known as STEC, which is short for "Shiga toxin-generating E. Coli."

One specially horrific strain, O157:H7, could make you very unwell. It motives belly cramps, vomiting, and bloody diarrhea. It's far the main purpose of acute kidney failure in youngsters.

Signs and symptoms and symptoms of E. Coli O157:H7 infection usually begin 3 or four days after publicity to the micro organism. However you could end up ill as fast as someday after publicity to greater than per week later. Signs and symptoms and signs and symptoms embody:

Diarrhea, which may additionally range from slight and watery to intense and bloody

Belly cramping, pain or tenderness

Nausea and vomiting, in a few humans

What does E. Coli appear like?

E. Coli is a rod-usual bacterium of the Enterobacteriaceae circle of relatives. It can stay in environments without or with air. These micro organism stay in the intestines of healthful people and warmth-blooded animals.

How many lines of E. Coli motive diarrhea?

Six one-of-a-kind traces of E. Coli are known to reason diarrhea. The ones lines are:

Shiga toxin-producing E. Coli (STEC): this is the micro organism maximum typically stated for E. Coli food infection. This stress is also called enterohemorrhagic E. Coli (EHEC) and verocytotoxin-generating E. Coli (VTEC).

Enterotoxigenic E. Coli (ETEC): This strain is generally referred to as a cause of vacationers' diarrhea.

Enteroaggregative E. Coli (EAEC).

Enteroinvasive E. Coli (EIEC).

Enteropathogenic E. Coli (EPIC).

Diffusely adherent E. Coli (DAEC).

How does E. Coli make you ill?

The most familiar strains of E. Coli that make you sick acquire this with the useful resource of manufacturing a toxin referred to as Shiga. This toxin damages the lining of your small intestine and motives your diarrhea. The ones traces of E. Coli also are referred to as Shiga toxin-producing E. Coli (STEC). The STEC that is most famous in North the us and most customarily said is E. Coli O157:H7, or really E. Coli O157

There are unique kinds of STEC which might be called non-O157 STEC. Those lines motive similar infection to the O157 pressure but are less probable to motive critical headaches.

Who can get inflamed with E. Coli?

Anyone who comes into contact with a disorder-inflicting stress of E. Coli can become infected. Those who are at first-rate danger are:

The very younger (newborns and children).

The elderly.

People who've weakened immune structures (for example, human beings with most cancers, diabetes, HIV, and girls who're pregnant).

Those who travel to certain countries.

Reasons

Just a few strains of E. Coli motive diarrhea. The E. Coli O157:H7 pressure belongs to a collection of E. Coli that produces a effective toxin that damages the liner of the small intestine. This could reason bloody diarrhea. You growth an E. Coli contamination whilst you ingest this pressure of bacteria.

Unlike many other sickness-causing bacteria, E. Coli can purpose an infection even in case you ingest best small quantities. Because of this, you may be sickened via way of E. Coli from ingesting a slightly undercooked hamburger or from swallowing a mouthful of infected pool water.

Capacity sources of publicity include contaminated meals or water and character-to-individual contact.

Infected food

The maximum common manner to get an E. Coli infection is by eating infected meals, at the side of:

Ground pork. While cattle are slaughtered and processed, E. Coli bacteria in their intestines can get at the red meat. Floor red meat combines meat from many special animals, increasing the danger of contamination.

Unpasteurized milk. E. Coli micro organism on a cow's udder or on milking device can get into uncooked milk.

CHAPTER TWO

Clean produce. Runoff from farm animals farms can contaminate fields wherein smooth produce is grown. Positive greens, together with spinach and lettuce, are specially liable to this form of contamination.

Infected water

Human and animal stool also can pollute ground and floor water, collectively with streams, rivers, lakes and water used to irrigate plants. Despite the fact that public water structures use chlorine, ultraviolet light or ozone to kill E. Coli, some E. Coli outbreaks were connected to inflamed municipal water components.

Personal water wells are a more purpose for

issue due to the fact many do now not have a way to disinfect water. Rural water assets are the maximum probable to be infected. A few people additionally were inflamed with E. Coli after swimming in swimming pools or lakes infected with stool.

Non-public contact

E. Coli bacteria can with out problems adventure from man or woman to character, especially even as infected adults and children do not wash their arms properly. Circle of relatives members of younger children with E. Coli infection are especially in all likelihood to get it themselves. Outbreaks have additionally came about among kids journeying petting zoos and in animal barns at county fairs.

How is an E. Coli infection diagnosed?

STEC infections are recognized via sending a pattern of your poop to a laboratory. Many labs can check for each STEC O157 and non-O157 STEC bacterial infections.

What steps are worried in getting a stool pattern to my healthcare provider?

Name your healthcare agency's workplace. They may have you are to be had for an place of job visit and give you a sterile stool collection cup and precise instructions to observe for a manner to accumulate a stool pattern. They will moreover email specific commands for gathering a sample at home.

Some desired commands for gathering a stool sample at domestic consist of:

First, wash your palms with cleaning soap and water.

If it's viable to urinate (pee) earlier than installing for the stool collection, do so. You don't want to get urine in your stool sample if you can help it.

To acquire diarrhea, tape a plastic bag to the rest room seat. You handiest want to acquire a small quantity – a couple tablespoons.

Location the plastic bag proper into a easy (washed and dried) plastic container and seal with lid.

Wash your palms with cleaning soap and water.

Write your name and date on the box, vicinity within some other bag, wash your palms another time and deliver on your healthcare provider at the equal day you gather your sample. If you can't deliver your sample right now, you could store it in your fridge for as much as 24 hours.

Do no longer collect the pattern from the relaxation room bowl. Do now not mixture in rest room paper, soap or water.

Whilst will i get the results once more from my stool pattern?

Most laboratories record again the outcomes within to 4 days. Your healthcare company will name you with the consequences as speedy as they come to be to be had or you'll be notified of your effects electronically if you have a web medical record set up along with your doctor or healthcare facility.

Treatments

The most effective manner your clinical health practitioner can understand for nice if you have an E. Coli infection is to send a sample of your stool to a lab to be analyzed.

Luckily, the contamination generally is going away on its personal.

For a few types of E.Coli related to diarrhea, along with the watery tourists' diarrhea, antibiotics can shorten the time period you have got signs and symptoms and signs and symptoms and might be utilized in reasonably immoderate instances.

But if you have fever or bloody diarrhea or in case your physician suspects Shiga toxin-generating E. Coli, antibiotics have to now not be taken. They are able to without a doubt increase the manufacturing of Shiga toxin and get worse your signs.

It's vital to rest and get masses of fluids to replace what your body is losing through vomiting or diarrhea.

Don't take over-the-counter medications that combat diarrhea. You don't want to sluggish down your digestive device, due to the fact that allows you to postpone your frame's dropping of the infection.

Whilst you begin to feel higher, maintain on with low-fiber components at the begin inclusive of:

Crackers

Toast

Eggs

Rice

Dairy products and food which may be excessive in fats or fiber may want to make your symptoms worse.

Chance factors

E. Coli will have an effect on all of us who is uncovered to the micro organism. But a few humans are more likely to increase issues than are others. Hazard factors encompass:

Age. Younger children and older adults are at higher danger of experiencing contamination due to E. Coli and more-vital complications from the contamination.

Weakened immune systems. Humans who've weakened immune systems — from AIDS or from pills to deal with maximum cancers or save you the rejection of organ transplants — are more likely to end up ill from ingesting E. Coli.

Ingesting effective kinds of food. Riskier food encompass undercooked hamburger; unpasteurized milk, apple juice or cider; and clean cheeses made from raw milk.

Time of 12 months. Although it is no longer clean why, the general public of E. Coli infections inside the U.S. Occur from June via September.

Decreased belly acid stages. Belly acid gives

a few safety toward E. Coli. If you take drug treatments to reduce stomach acid, which consist of esomeprazole (Nexium), pantoprazole (Protonix), lansoprazole (Prevacid) and omeprazole (Prilosec), you could increase your danger of an E. Coli infection.

Complications

Maximum wholesome adults get over E. Coli infection interior according to week. Some humans — particularly younger children and older adults — may additionally additionally expand a existence-threatening form of kidney failure referred to as hemolytic uremic syndrome.

CHAPTER THREE

Prevention

No vaccine or medicine can defend you from E. Coli-based completely infection, even though researchers are investigating potential vaccines. To lessen your risk of being exposed to E. Coli, avoid swallowing water from lakes or pools, wash your palms regularly, avoid risky components, and be careful for flow-contamination.

Volatile meals

Prepare dinner dinner hamburgers until they are one hundred sixty F (seventy one C). Hamburgers need to be well-completed, with out a crimson showing. But coloration isn't always a good manual to understand if the red meat is finished cooking. Meat — mainly if grilled — can brown before it's far absolutely cooked. Use a meat thermometer to make sure that meat is heated to as a minimum 160 F (71 C) at its thickest component.

Drink pasteurized milk, juice and cider. Any boxed or bottled juice saved at room temperature is in all likelihood to be pasteurized, despite the fact that the label does not say so. Keep away from any unpasteurized dairy products or juice.

Wash uncooked produce very well. Washing produce may not do away with all E. Coli — especially in leafy greens, which provide many locations for the micro organism to connect themselves to. Careful rinsing can remove dust and decrease the quantity of micro organism that can be clinging to the produce.

Wash utensils. Use warm soapy water on knives, counter tops and cutting forums in advance than and after they arrive into contact with easy produce or raw meat.

Preserve uncooked ingredients separate. This includes the usage of separate slicing boards for raw meat and foods, consisting of vegetables and fruits. In no way placed cooked hamburgers at the same plate you used for uncooked patties.

Wash your palms. Wash your hands after

getting geared up or ingesting food, using the toilet, or converting diapers. Make sure that kids also wash their arms in advance than eating, after the usage of the relaxation room and after touch with animals.

CONCLUSION

The best and best manner to avoid getting an E. Coli infection is to regularly wash your arms with cleaning soap and water. Wash your fingers earlier than and after managing foods (inclusive of prepping, cooking and serving food), after the use of the rest room, after touching animals (particularly farm or zoo animals), after converting diapers and after shaking arms or being touched thru others (you in no way recognize what their palms have touched). Washing your arms can not simplest save you contracting E. Coli, but moreover many distinctive infectious illness that are unfold from individual to person. Make not unusual hand washing a brand new habit.

Remember the fact that most lines of E. Coli are innocent. Even in case you do come down with the STEC O157 stress, your signs and signs and symptoms will remedy on their own inside five to seven days. Drink masses of fluids to live hydrated and get loads of relaxation.

Do name your healthcare issuer when you have diarrhea (and in particular bloody diarrhea) for greater than 3 days, have problem maintaining fluids down and function non-stop bouts of vomiting and have a fever. These symptoms may want to advocate you are developing excessive complications that would lead to kidney failure.

THE END